Table Of Contents

Chapter 1: Understanding the Sugar Trap

The Impact of Sugar on Your Body

Sugar is a pervasive ingredient in our modern diets, but its impact on our bodies can be detrimental. From weight gain to increased risk of chronic diseases like diabetes and heart disease, the effects of sugar consumption are far-reaching. Understanding how sugar affects your body is crucial for anyone looking to break the sugar habit and improve their health.

One of the most immediate impacts of sugar on your body is weight gain. When we consume sugar, our bodies quickly convert it into glucose, which is used for energy. However, excess glucose that is not immediately used is stored as fat, leading to weight gain over time. By reducing your sugar intake, you can help prevent this cycle of weight gain and work towards shedding pounds.

Furthermore, sugar consumption has been linked to inflammation in the body, which can contribute to a variety of health issues. Inflammation is the body's natural response to injury or infection, but chronic inflammation caused by a diet high in sugar can lead to conditions like arthritis, heart disease, and even cancer. By cutting back on sugar, you can reduce inflammation in your body and lower your risk of developing these chronic diseases.

Another major impact of sugar on your body is its effect on your blood sugar levels. When you consume sugar, your blood sugar levels spike, causing a surge of energy followed by a crash. This rollercoaster effect can leave you feeling tired, irritable, and craving more sugar to boost your energy levels again. By reducing your sugar intake, you can stabilize your blood sugar levels and avoid these energy crashes, leading to more consistent energy throughout the day.

In conclusion, the impact of sugar on your body is significant and far-reaching. From weight gain to inflammation to blood sugar fluctuations, reducing your sugar intake can have a positive impact on your overall health and well-being. By understanding how sugar affects your body and taking steps to break the sugar habit, you can improve your health, shed pounds, and feel better both physically and mentally.

Why Sugar is Addictive

Have you ever found yourself reaching for a sugary treat when you're feeling stressed or down? You're not alone. Sugar is a highly addictive substance that can wreak havoc on our bodies and minds. In this subchapter, we will explore why sugar is so addictive and how you can break free from its grip.

One reason sugar is so addictive is that it triggers the release of dopamine in the brain. Dopamine is a neurotransmitter that is associated with pleasure and reward. When we consume sugar, our brains release dopamine, making us feel good and reinforcing the desire to consume more sugar. This can create a cycle of cravings and overeating that can be hard to break.

Another reason sugar is addictive is that it can lead to a spike in blood sugar levels followed by a crash. When we consume sugary foods, our blood sugar levels rise rapidly, giving us a burst of energy. However, this energy is short-lived, and we soon experience a crash, leaving us feeling tired and irritable. This cycle can lead to cravings for more sugar to boost our energy levels again.

Sugar is also highly addictive because it can disrupt our hunger and satiety signals. When we consume sugary foods, our bodies release insulin to help regulate our blood sugar levels. However, consuming too much sugar can lead to insulin resistance, which can interfere with our body's ability to regulate hunger and satiety. This can lead to overeating and weight gain.

In addition to its addictive properties, sugar can also have negative effects on our health. Consuming too much sugar can lead to weight gain, diabetes, heart disease, and other chronic health conditions. By understanding why sugar is addictive, you can take steps to break free from its grip and improve your health and well-being.

In the next chapters of this book, we will explore practical strategies for detoxing from sugar and shedding pounds. By making small changes to your diet and lifestyle, you can break the sugar habit and achieve your health and weight loss goals. Remember, you are not alone in this journey, and with determination and support, you can overcome your sugar addiction and live a healthier, happier life.

Health Risks Associated with Excessive Sugar Consumption

Excessive sugar consumption can have a multitude of negative impacts on our health. One of the most immediate risks associated with consuming too much sugar is weight gain. Sugary foods and beverages are often high in calories and can contribute to an increase in body fat. This excess weight can lead to a host of health issues, including diabetes, heart disease, and even certain types of cancer. For those looking to shed pounds and improve their overall health, cutting back on sugar is a crucial first step.

In addition to weight gain, excessive sugar consumption can also lead to inflammation in the body. Chronic inflammation has been linked to a number of health conditions, including arthritis, asthma, and even Alzheimer's disease. By reducing our sugar intake, we can help to lower our risk of developing these inflammatory conditions and improve our overall well-being.

Another health risk associated with consuming too much sugar is an increased risk of developing type 2 diabetes. When we consume large amounts of sugar, our bodies can become resistant to insulin, the hormone that helps regulate blood sugar levels. Over time, this can lead to the development of diabetes, a serious and chronic condition that requires careful management. By cutting back on sugar, we can help to reduce our risk of developing this potentially life-threatening disease.

High sugar consumption has also been linked to an increased risk of heart disease. Diets high in sugar have been shown to raise levels of triglycerides, a type of fat found in the blood that can contribute to heart disease. Additionally, sugar can also increase levels of LDL cholesterol, the "bad" cholesterol that can clog arteries and lead to heart attacks and strokes. By reducing our sugar intake, we can help to protect our heart health and lower our risk of developing cardiovascular issues.

Overall, excessive sugar consumption poses a significant risk to our health and well-being. By making the decision to cut back on sugar and adopt a healthier diet, we can reduce our risk of weight gain, inflammation, diabetes, heart disease, and other serious health conditions. Breaking the sugar habit is not easy, but with determination and commitment, we can take control of our health and transform our lives for the better.

Chapter 2: Getting Started with Your Sugar Detox

Setting Clear Goals for Your Detox

Setting clear goals for your detox is essential in order to successfully break the sugar habit and shed pounds. Without clear objectives in mind, it can be easy to fall back into old patterns and sabotage your progress. By establishing specific and measurable goals, you can stay focused and motivated throughout the detox process.

The first step in setting clear goals for your sugar detox is to identify your reasons for wanting to eliminate sugar from your diet. Whether it's to lose weight, improve your overall health, or break free from sugar addiction, having a clear understanding of your motivation will help you stay committed when cravings strike. Write down your reasons for wanting to detox and keep them somewhere you can easily refer to when you need a reminder of why you started this journey.

Once you have identified your reasons for detoxing, it's time to set specific goals that align with your motivations. Whether you want to cut out all added sugars, reduce your overall sugar intake, or eliminate specific sugary foods from your diet, be sure to set clear and achievable goals that will help you stay on track. For example, you could set a goal to drink only water and herbal tea for beverages, or to avoid all sugary snacks and desserts for a set period of time.

In addition to setting specific goals for your sugar detox, it's important to establish a timeline for achieving them. Whether you want to detox for a week, a month, or longer, having a clear end date in mind can help you stay focused and motivated. Break down your goals into smaller, manageable steps and create a timeline for when you plan to achieve each one. This will help you stay accountable and track your progress throughout the detox process.

In conclusion, setting clear goals for your sugar detox is crucial for success. By identifying your motivations, setting specific and achievable goals, and establishing a timeline for achieving them, you can stay focused and committed to breaking the sugar habit and shedding pounds. Remember to be patient with yourself and celebrate your progress along the way. With dedication and perseverance, you can achieve your goals and set yourself on the path to a healthier, sugar-free lifestyle.

Cleaning Out Your Pantry

Cleaning out your pantry is an essential step in breaking the sugar habit and embarking on a successful detox journey. If you are someone who needs to stop consuming sugar in order to shed pounds and improve your overall health, taking a good look at what is lurking in your pantry is the first place to start.

Start by going through your pantry and reading labels carefully. Look for hidden sugars in items such as condiments, canned goods, and processed snacks. Ingredients like high fructose corn syrup, dextrose, and maltose are all forms of sugar that can sabotage your efforts to detox and lose weight. Be diligent in purging these items from your pantry to create a clean slate for your sugar-free journey.

Once you have identified and removed the sugary items from your pantry, it's time to restock with healthier alternatives. Fill your shelves with whole foods such as fruits, vegetables, nuts, seeds, lean proteins, and whole grains. These nutrient-dense foods will not only satisfy your hunger but also provide your body with the essential vitamins and minerals it needs to thrive without added sugars.

Organize your pantry in a way that makes healthy choices easy and accessible. Keep healthy snacks like pre-cut veggies, nuts, and seeds at eye level, while relegating sugary treats to the back of the pantry where they are out of sight and out of mind. By creating a space that supports your sugar detox goals, you are setting yourself up for success in breaking the sugar habit and losing weight.

Cleaning out your pantry is a crucial step in your journey to breaking the sugar habit and shedding pounds. By taking the time to remove sugary items, restock with healthier alternatives, and organize your pantry for success, you are setting yourself up for a successful sugar detox. Remember, a clean pantry is a clean start towards a healthier, sugar-free lifestyle.

Meal Planning for Success

Meal planning is a crucial aspect of successfully breaking the sugar habit and achieving weight loss goals. By carefully planning your meals in advance, you can ensure that you have healthy, sugar-free options readily available when hunger strikes. This can help prevent impulsive decisions to reach for sugary snacks or convenience foods that are high in added sugars.

When creating a meal plan for sugar detox and weight loss, it's important to focus on whole, nutrient-dense foods. This includes plenty of fruits, vegetables, lean proteins, and whole grains. These foods not only provide essential nutrients for your body but also help keep you feeling full and satisfied throughout the day.

One key aspect of meal planning for success is to always be prepared. This means having healthy snacks on hand, such as nuts, seeds, and cut-up vegetables, to prevent cravings for sugary treats. Additionally, planning your meals ahead of time can help you make healthier choices when dining out or ordering takeout, as you will already have a plan in place.

Another important tip for successful meal planning during a sugar detox is to keep things simple. Choose recipes that are easy to prepare and require minimal ingredients. This can help you stay on track with your goals without feeling overwhelmed by complicated meal plans or recipes.

By following these meal planning tips for success, you can take control of your sugar consumption, shed pounds, and improve your overall health. Remember that meal planning is a tool to help you reach your goals, so don't be afraid to experiment with different recipes and meal options to find what works best for you. With dedication and planning, you can break the sugar habit and achieve lasting weight loss success.

Chapter 3: Detoxifying Your Body

Eliminating Hidden Sugars

In our modern world, sugar seems to be hiding in almost everything we consume, from salad dressings to granola bars. These hidden sugars can wreak havoc on our health and make it incredibly difficult to shed those extra pounds. That's why it's crucial to learn how to identify and eliminate hidden sugars from our diets if we want to successfully break the sugar habit and lose weight.

One of the first steps in eliminating hidden sugars is to become a label detective. When shopping for groceries, take the time to carefully read the nutrition labels on packaged foods. Look for ingredients like high fructose corn syrup, dextrose, sucrose, and maltose, as these are all just different names for added sugars. By being mindful of these ingredients, you can start to make more informed choices about what you're putting into your body.

Another important strategy for eliminating hidden sugars is to cook more meals at home. When you prepare your own meals, you have complete control over the ingredients you use. This means you can avoid sneaky sources of sugar like store-bought sauces, marinades, and dressings. Instead, opt for whole, unprocessed foods and season them with herbs, spices, and other flavor enhancers that won't sabotage your sugar detox efforts.

It's also helpful to be aware of the different forms of sugar that can be found in foods. While it's easy to recognize the sweetness of table sugar, it's important to remember that sugars can also hide in less obvious forms like fruit juice concentrates and agave nectar. By educating yourself about the various types of sugars and their aliases, you can become more adept at spotting and avoiding hidden sugars in your diet.

By taking the time to educate yourself about hidden sugars and making conscious choices about what you eat, you can set yourself up for success on your sugar detox journey. Remember, breaking the sugar habit and shedding pounds is a process that requires patience and perseverance. But by prioritizing whole, unprocessed foods and learning to identify and eliminate hidden sugars, you can take control of your health and start to see real results in your weight loss efforts.

Incorporating Whole Foods into Your Diet

Incorporating Whole Foods into Your Diet is essential for anyone looking to break the sugar habit and shed pounds. Whole foods are nutrient-dense and provide your body with the essential vitamins and minerals it needs to function properly. By focusing on whole foods, you can avoid the added sugars and processed ingredients found in many packaged foods that can sabotage your weight loss efforts.

One of the best ways to incorporate whole foods into your diet is to focus on eating a variety of fruits and vegetables. These foods are packed with vitamins, minerals, and antioxidants that can help support your body's detoxification process and aid in weight loss. Try to fill half of your plate with fruits and vegetables at each meal to ensure you are getting a good balance of nutrients.

Whole grains are another important component of a healthy diet. Foods like brown rice, quinoa, and whole wheat bread are rich in fiber, which can help keep you feeling full and satisfied after meals. Additionally, the complex carbohydrates found in whole grains can provide a steady source of energy throughout the day, helping to curb sugar cravings.

Incorporating lean proteins into your diet is also important for breaking the sugar habit and shedding pounds. Foods like chicken, turkey, fish, and tofu are rich in protein, which can help support muscle growth and repair. Protein also helps to keep you feeling full and satisfied, reducing the likelihood of reaching for sugary snacks between meals.

Lastly, don't forget about healthy fats. Foods like avocados, nuts, seeds, and olive oil are rich in monounsaturated and polyunsaturated fats, which can help support heart health and keep you feeling satisfied. By incorporating a balance of whole foods into your diet, you can break the sugar habit, detox your body, and shed pounds for good.

Hydrating and Flushing Out Toxins

Hydrating plays a crucial role in the process of detoxifying your body from the harmful effects of sugar consumption. Drinking an adequate amount of water throughout the day helps to flush out toxins and waste products from your system, promoting overall health and well-being. Water is essential for proper digestion, nutrient absorption, and the elimination of waste products, which can become trapped in your body if you are dehydrated. By staying hydrated, you can support your body's natural detoxification processes and help to eliminate the build-up of toxins caused by excess sugar consumption.

In addition to drinking water, incorporating hydrating foods into your diet can also help to support your body's detoxification efforts. Foods such as cucumber, watermelon, and celery are high in water content and can help to keep you hydrated throughout the day. These foods also contain essential nutrients and antioxidants that can support your body's detoxification processes and promote overall health. By including hydrating foods in your diet, you can help to flush out toxins and waste products from your system, allowing your body to function at its best.

To further support your body's detoxification efforts, it is important to focus on eliminating sugary beverages and processed foods from your diet. These products are often high in sugar, artificial additives, and preservatives, which can contribute to the build-up of toxins in your body. By cutting back on these unhealthy foods and replacing them with hydrating, nutrient-rich options, you can support your body's natural detoxification processes and promote weight loss. Making small changes to your diet, such as swapping out soda for water or snacking on fresh fruits and vegetables instead of sugary treats, can have a significant impact on your overall health and well-being.

In addition to hydrating and flushing out toxins through diet and hydration, incorporating regular exercise into your routine can also support your body's natural detoxification processes. Physical activity helps to increase circulation, promote lymphatic drainage, and support the elimination of waste products from your body through sweat. By incorporating a mix of cardiovascular, strength training, and flexibility exercises into your routine, you can support your body's detoxification efforts, promote weight loss, and improve your overall health and well-being. Aim to engage in at least 30 minutes of moderate to vigorous exercise most days of the week to support your body's detoxification processes and help shed pounds.

In conclusion, hydrating and flushing out toxins are essential components of a successful sugar detox program. By staying hydrated, incorporating hydrating foods into your diet, eliminating sugary beverages and processed foods, and engaging in regular exercise, you can support your body's natural detoxification processes, promote weight loss, and improve your overall health and well-being. Making small, sustainable changes to your lifestyle can have a significant impact on your health and well-being, allowing you to break the sugar habit and achieve your weight loss goals.

Chapter 4: Managing Cravings and Withdrawal Symptoms

Identifying Triggers for Sugar Cravings

Understanding the root causes of your sugar cravings is essential in order to successfully break the habit and shed pounds. One of the first steps in this process is identifying the triggers that lead you to reach for sugary foods. By recognizing these triggers, you can begin to develop strategies to overcome them and reduce your consumption of sugar.

One common trigger for sugar cravings is stress. When we are feeling overwhelmed or anxious, our bodies often crave the quick energy boost that sugar provides. By finding healthier ways to cope with stress, such as exercise or meditation, you can reduce the urge to indulge in sugary treats.

Another trigger for sugar cravings is boredom. Many people turn to food, particularly sugary snacks, when they are feeling bored or restless. By finding alternative activities to occupy your time, such as reading a book or going for a walk, you can avoid the temptation to reach for sugar-laden foods.

Social situations can also be a trigger for sugar cravings. Whether it's a birthday party, office celebration, or dinner with friends, sugary treats are often readily available at social gatherings. By planning ahead and bringing your own healthy snacks, you can avoid the temptation to indulge in sugary foods and stay on track with your sugar detox goals.

Finally, certain foods and beverages can trigger sugar cravings as well. Foods high in refined carbohydrates, such as white bread and pasta, can cause blood sugar spikes and crashes that lead to cravings for sugar. Similarly, sugary beverages like soda and fruit juice can also contribute to cravings. By opting for whole foods and hydrating with water instead, you can reduce your overall sugar intake and break the cycle of cravings.

By identifying your personal triggers for sugar cravings and developing strategies to overcome them, you can successfully detox from sugar and achieve your weight loss goals. Remember, breaking the sugar habit is a journey, but with determination and perseverance, you can take control of your health and well-being.

Healthy Alternatives to Satisfy Your Sweet Tooth

For people that need to stop consuming sugar, finding healthy alternatives to satisfy your sweet tooth can be a game changer in your journey to break the sugar habit. While sugar cravings can be strong, there are plenty of natural and delicious options that can help you kick the sugar addiction and still enjoy a sweet treat.

One of the best ways to satisfy your sweet tooth without consuming refined sugar is to opt for fruits. Fruits are naturally sweet and packed with vitamins, minerals, and fiber. Whether you enjoy a juicy apple, a ripe banana, or some sweet berries, fruits can provide a satisfying sweetness without the negative effects of added sugars. Not only are fruits a healthier alternative, but they can also help curb sugar cravings and keep you feeling full and satisfied.

Another great option for satisfying your sweet tooth without the guilt is to indulge in dark chocolate. Dark chocolate contains less sugar than milk chocolate and is packed with antioxidants. Look for dark chocolate with a high cocoa content (at least 70%) to maximize the health benefits. Enjoy a square or two of dark chocolate as a treat when you're craving something sweet, and savor the rich flavor without the added sugar.

If you're looking for a quick and easy sweet fix, try making your own healthy desserts at home. There are plenty of recipes available that use natural sweeteners like honey, maple syrup, or stevia instead of refined sugar. From homemade fruit sorbets to chia seed puddings to avocado chocolate mousse, there are endless possibilities for creating delicious and nutritious treats that won't sabotage your sugar detox goals.

For those times when you're craving something cold and creamy, consider making your own smoothies or frozen treats. Blend up a refreshing smoothie with fresh fruits, leafy greens, and a splash of coconut water or almond milk for a sweet and satisfying drink. You can also freeze bananas or berries to make homemade "nice cream" – a healthy alternative to traditional ice cream that is just as delicious and satisfying.

By incorporating these healthy alternatives into your diet, you can satisfy your sweet tooth without compromising your sugar detox goals. Experiment with different flavors and ingredients to find what works best for you, and enjoy the benefits of breaking the sugar habit while still indulging in delicious treats. Remember, it's all about finding balance and making choices that support your health and well-being.

Coping Strategies for Withdrawal Symptoms

For people that need to stop consuming sugar, coping with withdrawal symptoms can be one of the biggest challenges on the journey to breaking the sugar habit. Withdrawal symptoms can include headaches, fatigue, irritability, and cravings for sugary foods. It's important to have coping strategies in place to help you navigate through these symptoms and stay on track with your sugar detox.

One coping strategy for managing withdrawal symptoms is to stay hydrated. Drinking plenty of water throughout the day can help flush out toxins from your body and alleviate some of the symptoms associated with sugar withdrawal. Additionally, staying hydrated can help curb cravings and keep you feeling more energized and focused.

Another helpful coping strategy is to focus on eating whole, nutrient-dense foods. By filling your plate with vegetables, fruits, lean proteins, and healthy fats, you can nourish your body and provide it with the nutrients it needs to function optimally. These foods can also help stabilize your blood sugar levels and reduce cravings for sugary treats.

Incorporating regular exercise into your routine can also be an effective way to cope with withdrawal symptoms. Exercise releases endorphins, which can help improve your mood and reduce feelings of irritability and fatigue. Additionally, physical activity can help distract you from cravings and provide a healthy outlet for stress and anxiety.

Lastly, finding support from others who are also on a sugar detox journey can be incredibly beneficial. Whether it's joining a support group, enlisting the help of a friend or family member, or working with a health coach, having someone to lean on during the tough moments can make a big difference. Remember, you're not alone in this journey, and there are plenty of resources available to help you successfully break the sugar habit and achieve your weight loss goals.

Chapter 5: Overcoming Challenges and Staying on Track

Dealing with Social Pressures and Temptations

Dealing with social pressures and temptations can be one of the biggest challenges when trying to break free from the sugar habit. Whether it's a birthday party, a night out with friends, or a holiday gathering, there always seems to be sugary treats lurking around every corner. But fear not, there are strategies you can employ to navigate these situations with ease and stay on track with your sugar detox journey.

First and foremost, it's important to communicate your goals with those around you. Let your friends and family know that you are trying to cut back on sugar and ask for their support. By sharing your intentions, you are more likely to receive encouragement and understanding, rather than pressure to indulge in sugary treats.

Another helpful tip is to come prepared. If you know you will be attending an event where sugary treats will be abundant, bring your own healthy snacks to munch on. This way, you won't feel deprived or left out, and you can still enjoy yourself without giving in to temptation.

It can also be helpful to have a game plan in place. Before heading into a potentially challenging situation, take a moment to visualize yourself successfully navigating the event without succumbing to sugary temptations. By mentally preparing yourself, you will be more likely to stay focused on your goals and resist the urge to indulge.

Finally, practice mindfulness and self-awareness. Pay attention to how your body feels before, during, and after consuming sugary treats. Take note of how certain foods make you feel and use that information to make healthier choices in the future. By being mindful of your body's signals, you can make more informed decisions about what you eat and ultimately break free from the sugar habit for good.

In conclusion, dealing with social pressures and temptations when trying to break the sugar habit can be challenging, but with the right strategies in place, it is entirely possible to stay on track and achieve your goals. By communicating your intentions, coming prepared, having a game plan, and practicing mindfulness, you can navigate any situation with ease and continue on your journey towards a healthier, sugar-free lifestyle.

Finding Support and Accountability

In order to successfully break the sugar habit and shed pounds, it is essential to find support and accountability. This can come in many forms, including seeking out a support group, enlisting the help of a friend or family member, or working with a health coach or nutritionist. Having someone to lean on during the challenging times can make all the difference in staying committed to your sugar detox journey.

Joining a support group specifically geared towards sugar detox can provide a sense of community and understanding that can be invaluable. These groups often offer resources, tips, and encouragement from others who are going through the same struggles. It can be comforting to know that you are not alone in your journey to break free from the grips of sugar addiction.

If joining a support group is not feasible, finding a friend or family member who can hold you accountable can also be effective. Whether it's checking in regularly to see how you are doing, providing encouragement, or even joining you in your sugar detox efforts, having someone by your side can make a significant difference in your success.

For those who prefer a more personalized approach, working with a health coach or nutritionist can provide tailored guidance and support throughout your sugar detox journey. These professionals can help you set realistic goals, create a personalized meal plan, and provide strategies for overcoming cravings and setbacks. Having someone to hold you accountable and provide expert advice can greatly increase your chances of success.

Ultimately, finding support and accountability is crucial for anyone looking to break the sugar habit and shed pounds. Whether it's joining a support group, enlisting the help of a friend or family member, or working with a health coach or nutritionist, having someone in your corner can make all the difference in achieving your goals. Don't be afraid to reach out for help – you don't have to do this alone.

Celebrating Your Successes and Progress

As you embark on your sugar detox journey to shed pounds and improve your health, it's important to take a moment to celebrate your successes and progress along the way. Breaking the sugar habit is no easy feat, and each step you take towards reducing your sugar intake is a victory worth celebrating. Whether you've successfully resisted the temptation of a sugary treat or made healthier choices at meal times, it's important to acknowledge and reward yourself for your efforts.

One way to celebrate your successes and progress is to set small, achievable goals for yourself along the way. For example, you could aim to reduce your daily sugar intake by a certain amount each week or incorporate more whole foods into your diet. By setting these mini goals and tracking your progress, you can see how far you've come and feel a sense of accomplishment with each milestone you reach.

Another way to celebrate your successes and progress is to treat yourself to non-food rewards. Instead of reaching for a sugary treat to celebrate, consider rewarding yourself with a new workout outfit, a massage, or a relaxing bath. These rewards can help reinforce positive behaviors and motivate you to continue making healthy choices on your sugar detox journey.

It's also important to celebrate the physical changes you may start to notice as a result of reducing your sugar intake. Whether you start to see changes in your weight, energy levels, or skin health, take the time to acknowledge these improvements and celebrate how far you've come. These visible changes can serve as motivation to continue on your sugar detox journey and achieve your weight loss goals.

In conclusion, celebrating your successes and progress on your sugar detox journey is an important part of staying motivated and focused on your goals. By setting small goals, rewarding yourself with non-food treats, and acknowledging the physical changes you experience, you can stay committed to breaking the sugar habit and shedding pounds for good. Remember to be kind to yourself and celebrate each step you take towards a healthier, sugar-free lifestyle.

Chapter 6: Maintaining a Sugar-Free Lifestyle

Strategies for Preventing Relapse

Relapsing into old habits can be one of the biggest challenges when it comes to breaking the sugar habit. However, with the right strategies in place, it is possible to prevent relapse and stay on track with your sugar detox journey. Here are some effective strategies for preventing relapse and successfully breaking the sugar habit for good.

The first strategy for preventing relapse is to identify and avoid triggers that may lead to cravings for sugar. This could include certain foods, social situations, or emotional cues that make you more likely to reach for sugary treats. By recognizing these triggers and finding alternative ways to cope with them, you can reduce the likelihood of giving in to cravings and relapsing.

Another important strategy for preventing relapse is to create a support system. Surround yourself with friends, family, or a support group who understand your goals and can offer encouragement and guidance when you are feeling tempted to indulge in sugar. Having a strong support system can make all the difference in staying committed to your sugar detox and avoiding relapse.

In addition to having a support system in place, it is important to have a plan for handling cravings when they arise. Instead of giving in to the urge to reach for sugary snacks, have healthier alternatives readily available, such as fruits, nuts, or vegetables. By having these options on hand, you can satisfy your cravings in a healthier way and avoid relapse.

Staying mindful and present in the moment is another key strategy for preventing relapse. By being aware of your thoughts, feelings, and actions, you can better understand why you may be tempted to consume sugar and make more conscious choices about what you eat. Mindfulness practices such as meditation, deep breathing, or journaling can help you stay focused on your goals and prevent relapse.

Lastly, it is important to celebrate your successes along the way. Breaking the sugar habit is a journey, and it is important to acknowledge and reward yourself for each milestone you reach. Whether it's treating yourself to a massage, buying a new outfit, or simply patting yourself on the back, celebrating your progress can help keep you motivated and prevent relapse. By implementing these strategies for preventing relapse, you can successfully break the sugar habit, detox your body, and shed pounds for good.

Creating a Sustainable and Balanced Diet

Creating a sustainable and balanced diet is essential for anyone looking to break their sugar habit and shed pounds. By incorporating a variety of nutrient-rich foods into your daily meals, you can ensure that your body is getting the necessary vitamins and minerals it needs to function optimally. A balanced diet consists of a combination of fruits, vegetables, whole grains, lean proteins, and healthy fats.

One of the first steps in creating a sustainable and balanced diet is to reduce or eliminate processed foods and sugary beverages from your daily intake. These items are often high in added sugars, which can contribute to weight gain and other health issues. Instead, focus on whole, natural foods that are rich in nutrients and low in added sugars. This will help to stabilize your blood sugar levels and reduce cravings for sugary treats.

In addition to cutting out processed foods and sugary beverages, it is important to incorporate a variety of fruits and vegetables into your diet. These foods are high in vitamins, minerals, and fiber, which can help to keep you feeling full and satisfied throughout the day. Aim to fill half of your plate with fruits and vegetables at each meal to ensure that you are getting a good balance of nutrients.

Lean proteins, such as chicken, fish, and tofu, are also essential for a balanced diet. Protein helps to build and repair tissue in the body, and can help to keep you feeling full and satisfied between meals. Try to include a source of lean protein in each meal to help stabilize your blood sugar levels and prevent cravings for sugary snacks.

Finally, don't forget to include healthy fats in your diet, such as avocados, nuts, and olive oil. These foods are important for brain health, hormone production, and nutrient absorption. By following these guidelines and creating a sustainable and balanced diet, you can successfully break your sugar habit and achieve your weight loss goals.

Incorporating Regular Physical Activity

Incorporating regular physical activity is essential when it comes to breaking the sugar habit and shedding pounds. Exercise not only helps to burn calories and boost metabolism, but it also plays a crucial role in regulating blood sugar levels and reducing cravings for sugary foods. By making physical activity a regular part of your routine, you can improve your overall health and well-being while making it easier to stick to your sugar detox plan.

One of the best ways to incorporate regular physical activity into your daily life is to find activities that you enjoy and that fit your schedule. Whether it's going for a brisk walk, taking a dance class, or hitting the gym, finding an exercise routine that you look forward to can make all the difference in staying motivated and committed to your sugar detox goals. Remember, the key is to start small and gradually increase the intensity and duration of your workouts as you build strength and endurance.

In addition to helping you break the sugar habit, regular physical activity can also help to combat stress and improve your mood. Exercise releases endorphins, which are known as "feel-good" hormones that can help to reduce anxiety and depression. By incorporating regular exercise into your routine, you can not only improve your physical health but also boost your mental and emotional well-being.

When it comes to incorporating regular physical activity into your sugar detox plan, it's important to set realistic goals and create a schedule that works for you. Whether you choose to exercise in the morning before work, during your lunch break, or in the evening after dinner, finding a time that fits your lifestyle and preferences will make it easier to stick to your routine. Remember, consistency is key when it comes to seeing results, so make a commitment to yourself to prioritize your health and well-being by making exercise a non-negotiable part of your day.

Overall, incorporating regular physical activity into your sugar detox plan is essential for breaking the sugar habit and shedding pounds. By finding activities that you enjoy, setting realistic goals, and creating a schedule that works for you, you can make exercise a regular part of your routine and reap the many benefits that come with staying active. Remember, staying committed to your fitness goals will not only help you achieve success in your sugar detox journey but also improve your overall health and well-being in the long run.

Chapter 7: Shedding Pounds and Reaping the Benefits

Monitoring Your Progress and Adjusting Your Goals

As you embark on your sugar detox journey to lose weight, it is essential to monitor your progress along the way. Keeping track of your daily sugar intake, weight loss, and overall well-being will help you stay on track and make necessary adjustments to your goals. One way to monitor your progress is by keeping a daily food journal where you can log everything you eat and drink. This will give you a clear picture of how much sugar you are consuming and help you identify any patterns or triggers that may be causing you to reach for sugary treats.

In addition to tracking your food intake, it is important to regularly weigh yourself and take measurements of your body. This will help you see the physical changes that are occurring as a result of your sugar detox efforts. Remember that weight loss is not the only indicator of progress, so pay attention to how your clothes fit and how you feel overall. If you notice any positive changes in your energy levels, mood, or sleep patterns, celebrate these non-scale victories as well.

As you monitor your progress, be prepared to adjust your goals as needed. If you find that you are not seeing the results you hoped for, consider revisiting your initial goals and making them more specific, measurable, and achievable. For example, instead of just aiming to "cut back on sugar," set a goal to limit your daily sugar intake to a certain number of grams. This will give you a clearer target to work towards and make it easier to track your progress.

It is also important to be flexible and willing to make changes to your goals as you learn more about what works best for your body. If you find that a particular approach is not yielding the results you want, don't be afraid to try something new. Experiment with different meal plans, exercise routines, and stress management techniques to see what helps you feel your best and support your weight loss goals.

By monitoring your progress and adjusting your goals along the way, you will be better equipped to stay motivated and committed to your sugar detox journey. Remember that this is a process, and it's okay to make mistakes or experience setbacks. Stay focused on your ultimate goal of breaking the sugar habit and shedding pounds, and celebrate each small victory along the way.

Recognizing Non-Scale Victories

In the journey to break free from sugar addiction and shed pounds, it's important to recognize and celebrate non-scale victories along the way. While stepping on the scale can be a helpful tool to track progress, it's not the only measure of success when it comes to overcoming sugar cravings and achieving a healthier lifestyle. Non-scale victories are the small, but significant achievements that can motivate and inspire you to keep going on your sugar detox journey.

One example of a non-scale victory could be having more energy throughout the day. When you cut out sugar from your diet, you may find that you no longer experience the mid-afternoon crash or feel sluggish in the mornings. This newfound energy can help you be more productive at work, have more focus during workouts, and overall feel more vibrant and alive.

Another non-scale victory to celebrate is improved skin health. Many people who consume high amounts of sugar often experience acne breakouts or dull, lackluster skin. By eliminating sugar from your diet, you may notice clearer, brighter skin that glows from within. This can boost your confidence and make you feel more comfortable in your own skin.

A non-scale victory that often goes unnoticed is improved mental clarity and focus. Sugar can have a negative impact on cognitive function, leading to brain fog and difficulty concentrating. By detoxing from sugar, you may find that your mental clarity improves, making it easier to stay focused at work, remember important tasks, and make better decisions throughout the day.

One of the most rewarding non-scale victories is increased self-confidence and self-esteem. As you make healthier choices and break free from sugar addiction, you'll start to feel more confident in your ability to take control of your health and make positive changes in your life. This newfound self-assurance can spill over into other areas of your life, leading to improved relationships, career success, and overall happiness.

In conclusion, recognizing and celebrating non-scale victories is essential for anyone looking to break the sugar habit and lose weight. These small wins can help keep you motivated, inspired, and on track to achieving your health goals. So, next time you resist a sugary temptation, notice an improvement in your energy levels, or feel more confident in your own skin, take a moment to celebrate these non-scale victories and pat yourself on the back for all the hard work you've put in.

Embracing a New, Healthier Version of Yourself

Embarking on a sugar detox journey is not just about cutting out sugar from your diet. It's about embracing a new, healthier version of yourself - both physically and mentally. Breaking the sugar habit is not easy, but with dedication and commitment, you can achieve a healthier lifestyle and shed those unwanted pounds.

One of the first steps in embracing a new, healthier version of yourself is to understand the impact sugar has on your body. Sugar is highly addictive and can lead to weight gain, inflammation, and a host of other health issues. By detoxing from sugar, you are taking control of your health and well-being. You are choosing to prioritize your health over the temporary pleasure that sugar provides.

As you begin your sugar detox journey, it's important to focus on nourishing your body with whole, nutrient-dense foods. This means incorporating plenty of fruits, vegetables, lean proteins, and healthy fats into your diet. These foods will help stabilize your blood sugar levels, reduce cravings, and provide your body with the essential nutrients it needs to thrive.

In addition to focusing on nutrition, it's also important to prioritize self-care during your sugar detox. This means getting enough sleep, managing stress, and engaging in regular physical activity. Taking care of yourself holistically will not only support your detox efforts but also help you feel more energized, focused, and motivated to stick to your goals.

Embracing a new, healthier version of yourself is a journey that requires patience, perseverance, and self-compassion. By committing to breaking the sugar habit, you are taking a powerful step towards improving your health, losing weight, and reclaiming control of your life. Remember, you are capable of achieving your goals and becoming the best, healthiest version of yourself.

Chapter 8: Conclusion

Reflecting on Your Journey

As you embark on your journey to break the sugar habit and detox your body, it is important to take some time to reflect on how you got to this point. For many of us, sugar has become a crutch, a way to cope with stress, boredom, or emotions. It is essential to understand the role that sugar has played in your life and how it has affected your health and well-being.

Take a moment to think about the reasons why you want to stop consuming sugar. Is it to lose weight, improve your overall health, or simply to have more energy and feel better? Whatever your motivation may be, it is crucial to keep it at the forefront of your mind as you navigate the challenges of breaking the sugar habit.

Reflect on your past attempts to cut back on sugar or detox your body. What worked well for you? What obstacles did you face? By examining your past experiences, you can identify patterns and behaviors that may have contributed to your sugar consumption. Use this knowledge to make informed decisions and set realistic goals for yourself moving forward.

Consider keeping a journal to track your progress and reflect on your daily experiences. Write down how you feel physically and emotionally when you consume sugar versus when you avoid it. Document any cravings, triggers, or setbacks you encounter along the way. This journal can serve as a powerful tool for self-reflection and help you stay accountable to your goals.

Remember, breaking the sugar habit is a journey, not a destination. It is normal to have ups and downs, good days and bad days. Be gentle with yourself and celebrate your successes, no matter how small they may seem. By reflecting on your journey and staying committed to your goals, you can overcome the grip that sugar has on your life and achieve lasting health and wellness.

Tips for Long-Term Success

In order to achieve long-term success in breaking the sugar habit and shedding pounds, it is important to implement a few key tips and strategies. The first tip is to gradually reduce your sugar intake instead of trying to quit cold turkey. This will help ease the withdrawal symptoms and make the process more manageable. Start by cutting out sugary drinks and snacks, and gradually eliminate other sources of added sugars from your diet.

Another important tip for long-term success is to focus on whole, unprocessed foods. This means eating plenty of fruits, vegetables, lean proteins, and whole grains. These foods are not only nutrient-dense, but they also help stabilize blood sugar levels and reduce cravings for sugary treats. Make sure to plan your meals ahead of time and have healthy snacks on hand to avoid temptation.

In addition, it is crucial to stay hydrated throughout the day. Drinking plenty of water can help curb cravings for sugar and keep you feeling full between meals. Aim to drink at least eight glasses of water a day, and consider adding herbal teas or infused water for added flavor without the added sugars.

It is also important to get moving and incorporate regular exercise into your routine. Exercise not only helps burn calories and promote weight loss, but it also boosts mood and reduces stress – two common triggers for sugar cravings. Find an activity that you enjoy, whether it's walking, jogging, yoga, or weight training, and make it a priority in your daily schedule.

Finally, remember that breaking the sugar habit is a journey, not a destination. It's okay to slip up occasionally or indulge in a sweet treat every now and then. The key is to learn from these moments and get back on track as soon as possible. By implementing these tips for long-term success, you can break the sugar habit, shed pounds, and create a healthier, happier lifestyle for yourself.

Continuing Your Health and Wellness Journey

Congratulations on taking the first step towards breaking free from the sugar habit and embarking on your health and wellness journey. As you continue on this path, it is important to remember that this is a process, not a quick fix. In order to truly detox from sugar and shed pounds, it is essential to make long-term lifestyle changes that will support your overall health and well-being.

One key aspect of continuing your health and wellness journey is to focus on nourishing your body with whole, nutrient-dense foods. This means filling your plate with plenty of fruits, vegetables, lean proteins, and healthy fats. These foods will not only help to keep you full and satisfied, but they will also provide your body with the essential nutrients it needs to function optimally.

In addition to eating a balanced diet, it is important to stay hydrated by drinking plenty of water throughout the day. Water helps to flush out toxins from your body and keep your organs functioning properly. It is also important to limit your intake of sugary beverages, such as soda and fruit juice, as they can sabotage your efforts to detox from sugar.

Another important aspect of continuing your health and wellness journey is to engage in regular physical activity. Exercise not only helps to burn calories and support weight loss, but it also has numerous other health benefits, including improved mood, increased energy, and reduced risk of chronic diseases. Find activities that you enjoy, whether it's going for a walk, taking a fitness class, or practicing yoga, and make them a regular part of your routine.

Lastly, it is important to remember that progress is not always linear. There may be times when you slip up and indulge in sugary treats, but it's important to not get discouraged. Instead, use these slip-ups as learning opportunities and recommit to your health and wellness goals. By staying focused, consistent, and patient, you will be able to break the sugar habit, detox your body, and shed pounds for good.